Penguin Books

THE DESPERATE WOMAN'S GUIDE TO THERAPY

GW00732703

A mid-century product of Tyneside, Jo Nesbitt went to a convent school, then London University, where the college shrink interpreted the giant nuns which frequented her dreams as 'phallic symbols', an insight which she has always treasured. She has freelanced since 1978, and her work has appeared in *Time Out*, the *New Statesman*, *Spare Rib*, *Open University* and many educational publications. After moving to Holland in 1981, she published four books, of which *The Modern Ladies' Compendium* (cartoons) and *The Great Escape of Doreen Potts* (for children) also appeared in English.

Born Disgusted in Tunbridge Wells during the Second World War, Gillian Reeve had no choice but to be a subversive. Educated at London University, she has worked for campaigning organizations and as a freelance journalist and writer. She has co-authored two books, including *Offence of the Realm: How Peace Campaigners Get Bugged*, and has had three plays broadcast on BBC Radio 4. A resident of north London, she attended a seminal three-year course on psychoanalysis and female identity and is active in the medical peace movement and on the couch.

The Desperate Woman's Guide to Therapy

Text by Gillian Reeve
Drawings by Jo Nesbitt

Penguin Books

PENGUIN BOOKS

Published by the Penguin Group
Penguin Books Ltd, 27 Wrights Lane, London W8 5TZ, England
Penguin Books USA Inc., 375 Hudson Street, New York, New York 10014, USA
Penguin Books Australia Ltd, Ringwood, Victoria, Australia
Penguin Books Canada Ltd, 10 Alcorn Avenue, Toronto, Ontario, Canada M4V 3B2
Penguin Books (NZ) Ltd, 182–190 Wairau Road, Auckland 10, New Zealand

Penguin Books Ltd, Registered Offices: Harmondsworth, Middlesex, England

Published by Penguin Books 1997
10 9 8 7 6 5 4 3 2 1

Text copyright © Gillian Reeve, 1997
Drawings copyright © Jo Nesbitt, 1997
All rights reserved

The moral right of the authors has been asserted

Typeset in Monotype Photina
Printed in England by Clays Ltd, St Ives plc

Except in the United States of America, this book is sold subject
to the condition that it shall not, by way of trade or otherwise, be lent,
re-sold, hired out, or otherwise circulated without the publisher's
prior consent in any form of binding or cover other than that in
which it is published and without a similar condition including this
condition being imposed on the subsequent purchaser

For all the therapists we have loved, hated and dated ...

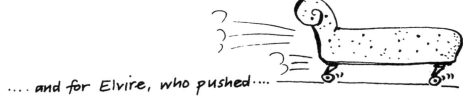

.... and for Elvire, who pushed ....

Contents

Why Go into Therapy?   1

Choosing a Therapist   7

Surviving the First Session   21

Some Common Terms and Techniques   31

Difficult Stages to Get Through   77

Reaching the Terminus   101

Some Alternatives to Therapy   115

Why Go into Therapy?

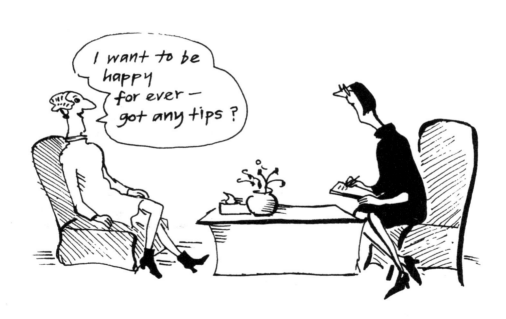

Therapy involves self-discovery. This may at times be painful, but can also be fun, and should ultimately be liberating.

Most women go into therapy because they have suffered a crisis, or are depressed, or feel their life is blocked in some way. Or there may be a more specific reason:

You can't leave the house.

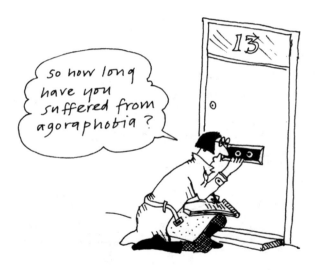

Going off sex for no good reason.
If you have a good reason, you
might be better off in a convent
– it would certainly be cheaper.

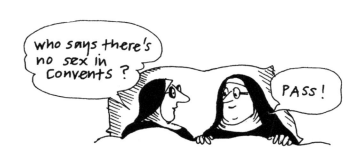

Friends may have hinted...

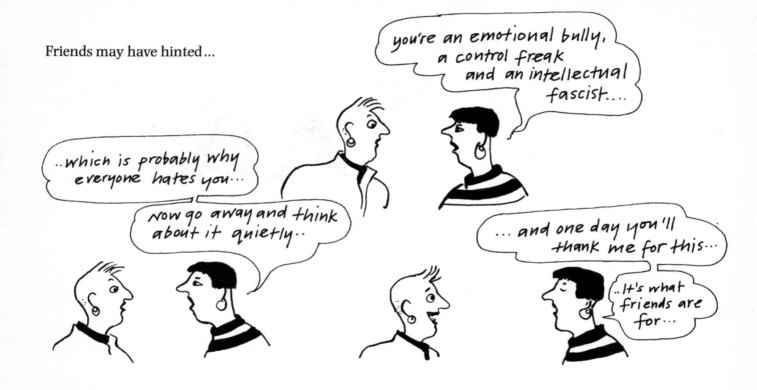

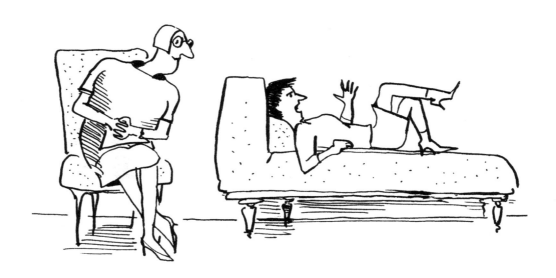

Your partner suggests marriage or is constantly leaving. Or you can't find a partner.

You want to be IT for someone for 50 minutes on a regular basis.

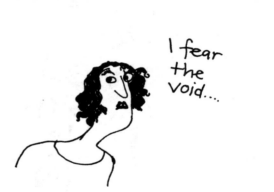

I fear
the
void....

Choosing a Therapist

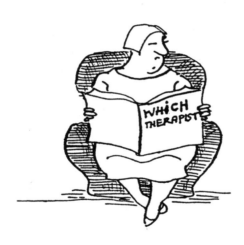

First, you need to decide whether you're looking for a long-term relationship or a short-term fix for a specific problem.

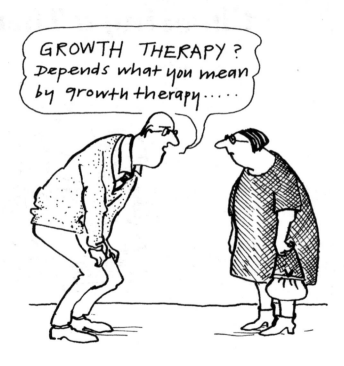

You don't have to go to the first therapist you find. If in doubt, check their credentials. If these comprise having done a three-month correspondence course in hypnosis in 1975, or having been brought up in an attic opposite the Freud Museum, better try elsewhere.

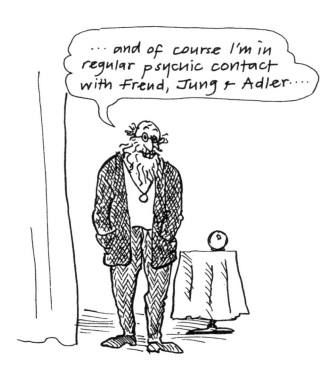

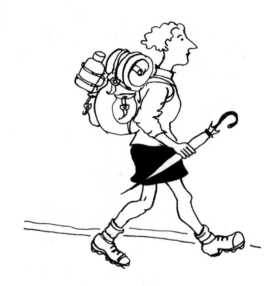

It's as well to choose someone
who lives close by, or is at least
easily accessible. Otherwise
you may spend your whole day
travelling.

If she can offer you a session only at six in the morning and you normally get up at nine, give that one a miss.

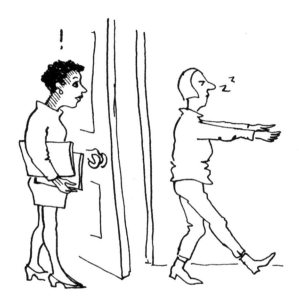

If you feel you want to see a woman, a man in his sixties is unlikely to be able to do much for you. On the other hand, it's as well not to have too much in common with your therapist.

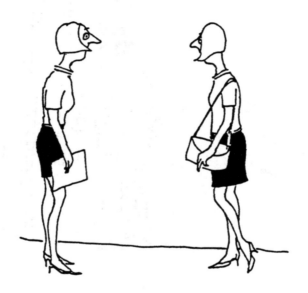

It's always wise to have a preliminary interview. For one thing, you can check out comfort and privacy. Beware of eavesdroppers – or noises in the next room.

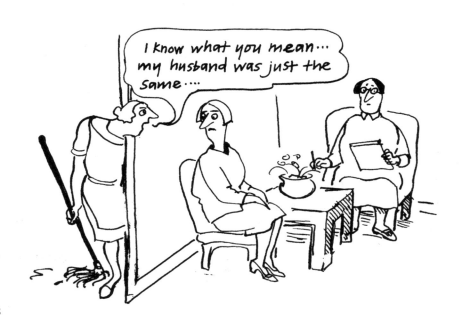

What am I? This is an existential question that needs to be answered as soon as you set foot in the door.

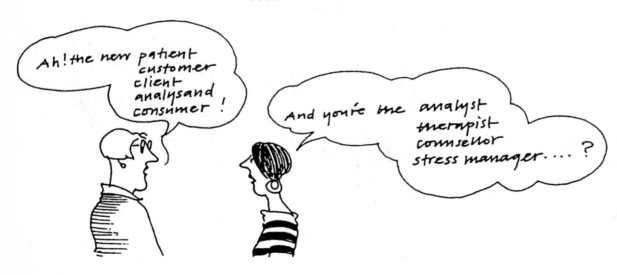

How do you feel about the therapist's taste in clothes? Can you bear to sit or even lie at close quarters to long silk scarves and dangling earrings? What about shrunken grey trousers, check pullovers and yellow socks?

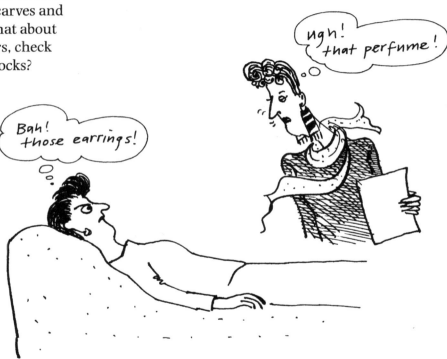

You will need to negotiate payment. You may resent the fee demanded, which could be up to ten times what many women earn in an hour. Are you strong enough to bargain? If so, perhaps you don't need the therapy after all. If not, you may have to resign yourself to several sessions working out why you didn't.

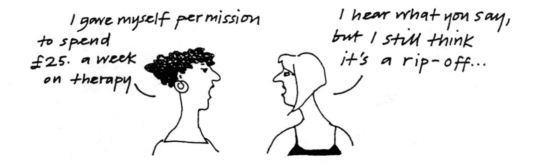

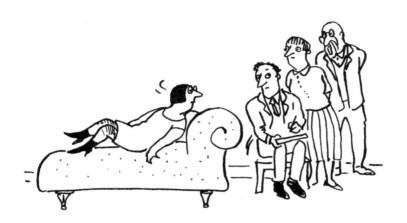

Some therapists, especially younger ones, work under the supervision of more experienced colleagues. You may want to ask whether the therapist is in such a system. Some people find the idea of supervision reassuring. Others don't like to think of themselves being a 'case' to be discussed with other professionals.

Whichever type of therapy you choose, most people now agree that it is the relationship between therapist and client that is the key to success. So in the end it will probably come down to a gut feeling. Do you trust and feel safe with this person?

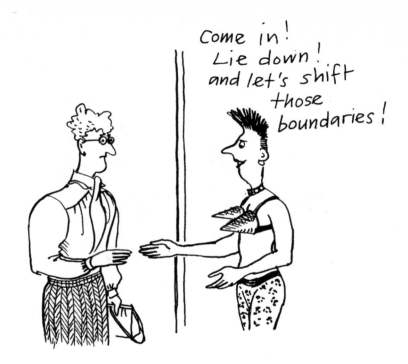

There are over 50,000 therapists
in the UK, and though it may
seem that most of them live in
north London, many have in fact
already headed for the hills. So
the chances are that, wherever
you live, someone, somewhere,
will be right for you.

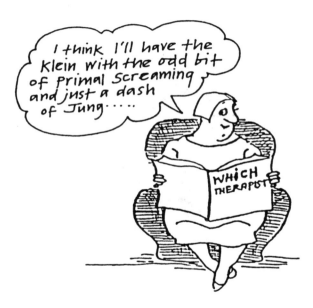

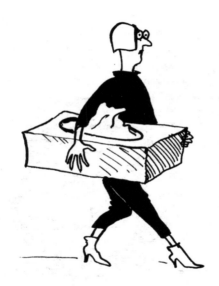

Surviving the First Session

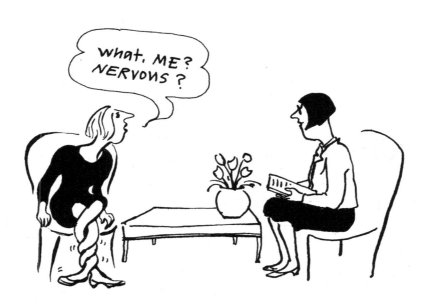

The first session is likely to be full of pitfalls.

First, you have to negotiate where you sit. You may be asked to choose between the couch and the chair. Would the couch make you too vulnerable or passive? Will you drop off to sleep? Suppose it squeaks? What if there are cat hairs on the pillow that will bring out your allergy or get on your clothes?

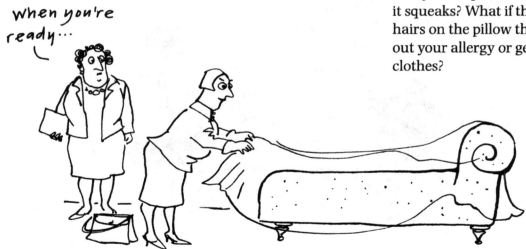

when you're ready...

Freud used a couch, he said, 'because I cannot put up with being stared at by other people for eight hours or more a day'. Also he didn't want his expressions to influence his patients.

If you choose the chair, it means you have to spend the next 50 minutes looking this stranger in the eye. You may even have to face the horror of finding a wet Kleenex in some deep recess.

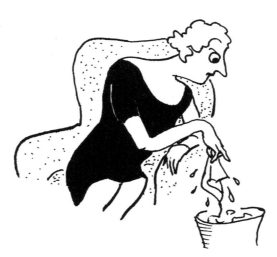

Be prepared for a massive clothes crisis. Padded shoulders will give a very different message from a low-cut dress or a floral outfit. If you're going in for one of the more exotic types of therapy, it's as well not to wear a tight skirt in case you're offered a cushion on the floor or a waterbed.

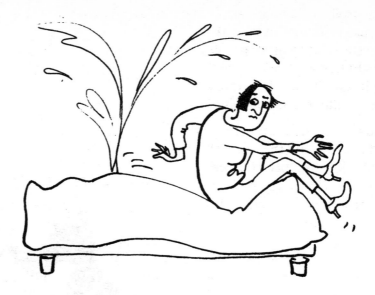

You may find it difficult to choose an opening gambit. Should you comment on the therapist's daffodils? Do you recount yesterday's events in minute detail? Or do you go for the jugular, and recall how at an early age you came upon your mother strangling a pheasant?

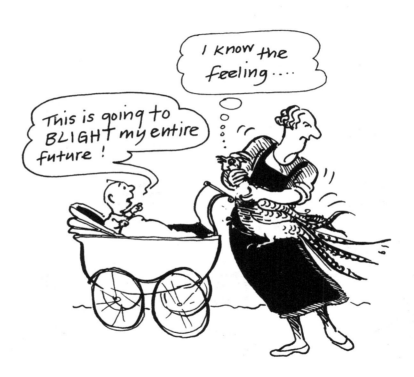

There is a strong chance that at some point you'll be struck dumb. An extended silence can feel like a valuable time for reflection – or a terrible waste of money.

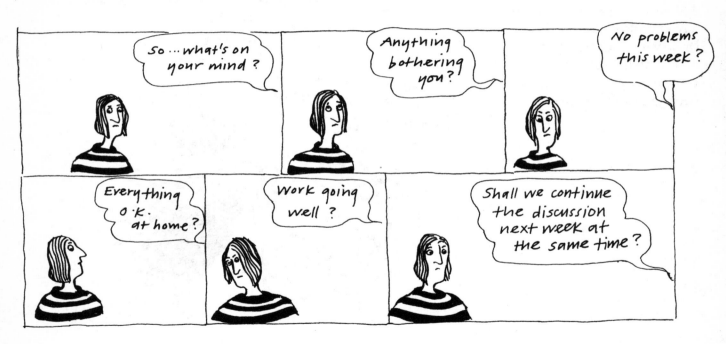

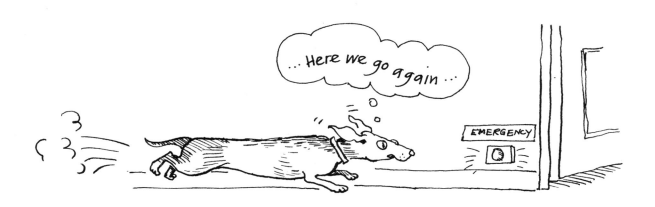

Alternatively, you may not be
able to let the therapist get a
word in edgeways. One client
was cut short by her therapist's
dachshund running in: was this
a secret sign?

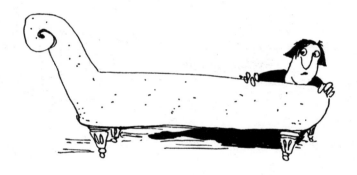

You may find the unconditional
positive regard a little daunting.

If you express an opinion that the therapist's plants need watering, or even feeding, this will certainly be analysed.

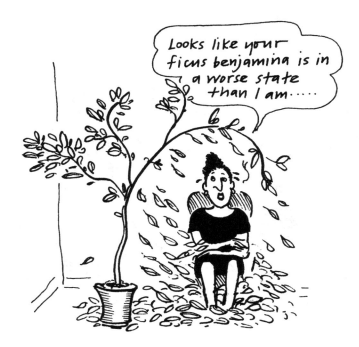

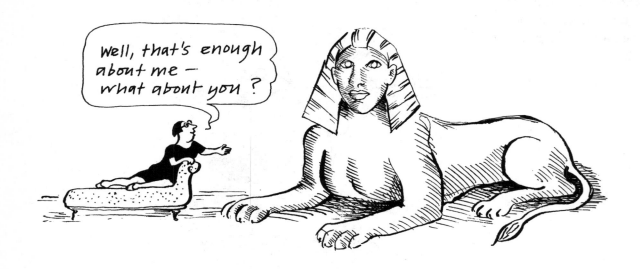

Some Common Terms and Techniques

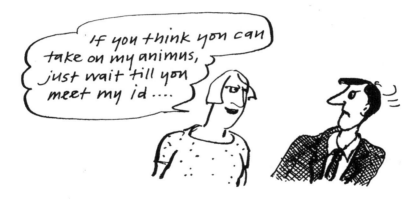

Therapy is a complex business. Each school of thought has its own theory, style and language. The more classical types tend to work with the unconscious, with the therapist keeping a distance and using interpretation to help uncover problems.

More recently developed therapies tend to assume the client knows which problems are crucial, and work with what she presents. But in most types, it is now being realized, the techniques are remarkably similar.

Short-term methods of therapy are usually concerned with relieving abnormal and distressing behaviour such as animal phobias.

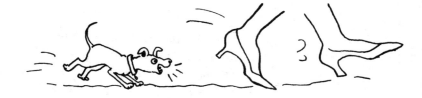

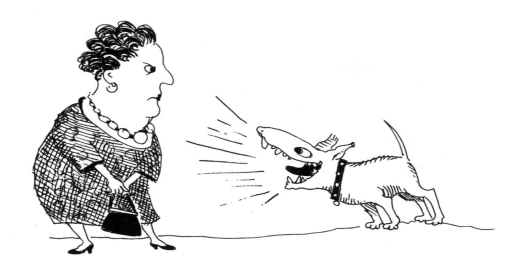

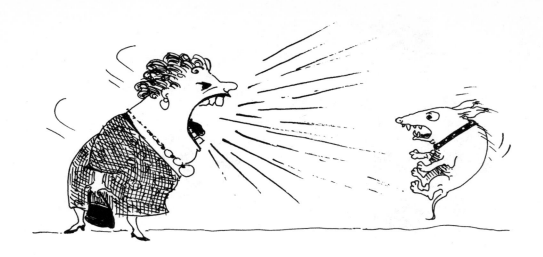

Some Classical Therapies

Freudian

Sigmund Freud was the pioneer of psychoanalysis. His unique and revolutionary contribution to mental health was to develop the 'talking cure'. By analysing distressing symptoms and exploring the unconscious material of his patients through free association, slips of the tongue and dreams, he aimed to help them overcome their resistance to self-knowledge and bring emotional release. All modern psychotherapeutic treatments are based to some extent on his discoveries.

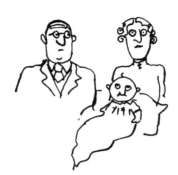

Freud is best known for pointing out the significance of infantile sexuality. This, he thought, culminated in the 'Oedipus complex', in which every child unconsciously both desires and feels rejected by its parents.

Unfortunately, the popular misconception that everyone going into therapy will be accused of having fallen in love with their mother or father has put a lot of people off.

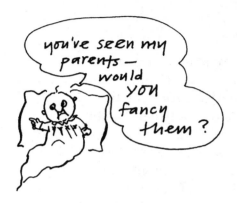

Freud used the term 'id' to describe the instinctual drives – the innate source of human motivation. His admission that he didn't actually know what women wanted, and feminist agreement with this, led to a radical rethink of the Oedipus complex.

WAS **WILL** das **WEIB?**

Jungian

Carl Gustav Jung split from Freud and psychoanalysis to develop his own system of analytical psychology. His experience of the spiritual aspects of life convinced him that there was a part of the unconscious deeper than the personal layer. This he named the collective unconscious, believing it common to all mankind and revealed as images in dreams, fairy tales and religions, and in the mythologies of different cultures at different periods of history. He called these common images 'archetypes'.

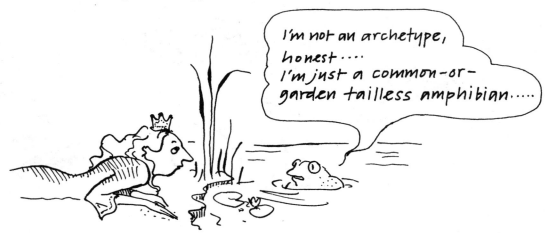

I'm not an archetype, honest....
I'm just a common-or-garden tailless amphibian.....

One archetype is the good or bad mother figure (goddess or witch) which underlies the experience of an actual mother. Another is the 'shadow', a way of describing unrecognized or unacknowledged parts of the personality. Jung also believed each individual has an unconscious contrasexual persona which possesses certain attributes of the opposite sex – in women this is called the 'animus', in men the 'anima'.

A Jungian analysis is particularly suitable for mid-life onwards. The analyst aims to assist the process of individuation – achieving integration and self-fulfilment – by actively engaging with you, to enable a greater sense of choice and creativity.

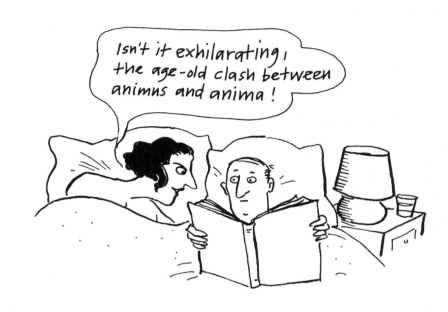

Kleinian

A Kleinian analysis will take you back to the earliest years of your life. Melanie Klein developed her theories by using new techniques to psychoanalyse very young children. She found the infant's inner world full of rampant desires and fantasies. These interacted with the external world, such as its mother's breast – which it experienced as good and loved if accessible, bad and hated if not.

This caused feelings of anxiety due to guilt and fear of loss, as well as sadistic impulses, destructive aggression and fear of retaliation. At other times it led to envy or gratitude. Here lay the origins of ambivalence.

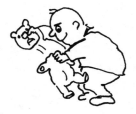

40

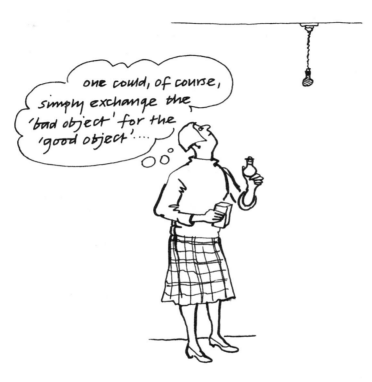

A Kleinian analyst considers changing a lightbulb.....

Klein's discoveries of these primitive layers of the mind have been influential in much of adult analysis. But she has been criticized for putting too much stress on the inner world and too little on the impact of real events. For instance, a patient who arrives with some physical problem may receive no comment from her analyst, tempting her to go straight home.

A Kleinian analysis usually takes place three or more times a week and may continue for many years.

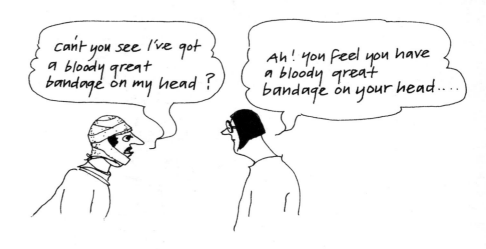

Using Dreams

In most types of therapy dreams are considered significant, though the way they are worked with and made sense of varies.

Freud believed dreams were 'the royal road to the unconscious'. The visual images have a symbolic meaning which can be interpreted to achieve an understanding of what they represent.

But problems may arise for people who claim they never dream, or can't remember their dreams when they wake up.

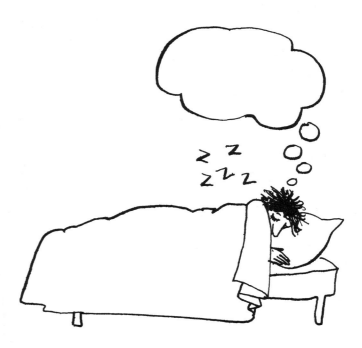

How to catch your dreams: some hints

When you go to bed, allow for a period of relaxation before you fall asleep. Cocoa may help. Keep pencil and paper or tape recorder handy by the bed.

When you wake up, don't move. Then write or record whatever you remember and feel straight away, before any bedfellows such as partners or pets can distract you. There is nothing more likely to scare off a significant dream than an urgent demand for breakfast.

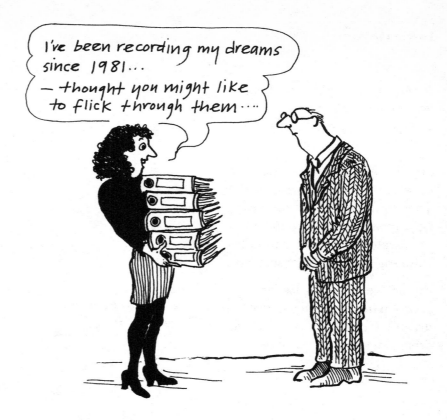

A test in dream interpretation:

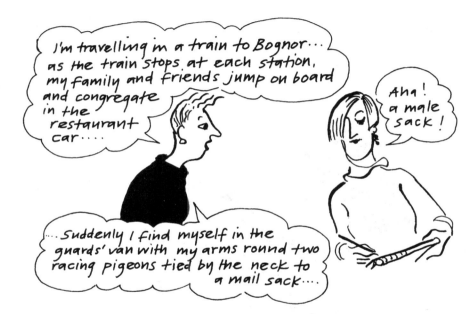

The patient continues: 'I'm crooning to them and comforting them. The guard arrives and looks pretty surprised to see me. His hair looks just like yours. He tries to take my hand, but I avoid him and untie the pigeons. The next thing I know I'm driving the train...'

The answer is that there's no correct answer. If the interpretation feels right for you, it's valid.

Some Common Terms

Projection

If you are late and feel that your therapist is angry with you, it's more likely that you are angry with your therapist. Attributing your feelings to someone else happens all the time, and therapy is the ideal time to discover when and why you do this.

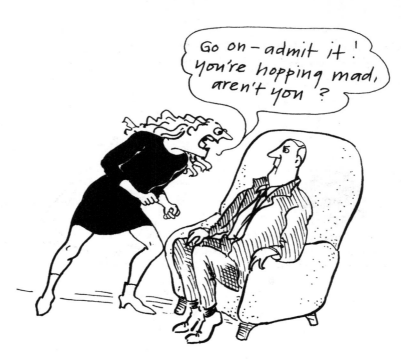

Introjection

Do you feel there is often some-one on your shoulder checking you are doing the right thing? If so, you've taken in (introjected) the ideas, beliefs or attitudes of important people in your life such as your parents.

Therapy will aim to find out who these internalized beings are and help you get away from them.

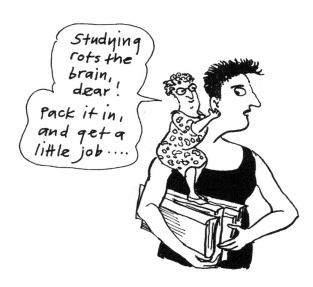

Transference

You will sometimes relate to your therapist as though she were a significant person from your early life such as a parent, brother or sister. Analysing this process step by step should bring you nearer to experiencing and understanding your present feelings and conflicts.

Transference also happens in everyday relationships, of course, and can account for people getting involved with highly unsuitable others.

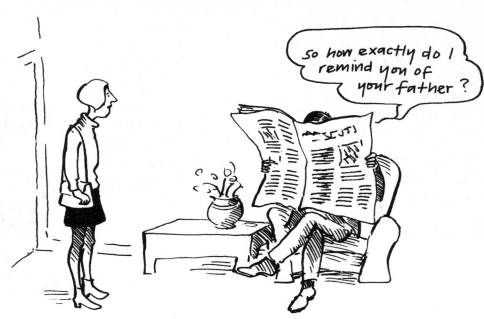

Countertransference

How the therapist feels about you will give an important clue as to the reactions you get from others. For example, if she yawns a lot, you may be fundamentally boring. What she has to do is to distinguish between her own feelings, the reactions which come from her own past experiences, and reactions which you evoke. This is the point at which she really earns her money.

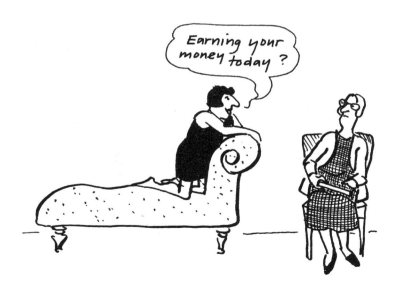

Displacement

If you continually fall in love with men who resemble your father, you're exhibiting the neurotic defence mechanism of displacement.

Sublimation

This is considered to be a more mature form of displacement. For instance, you may sublimate your need for sex into playing tennis, or playing the viola, or writing novels – or therapy.

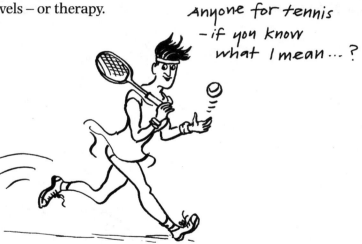

Reaction formation

If you feel a sudden desire to sit on your therapist's lap, and instead dive under the couch, this is reaction formation. It's doing the complete opposite of what you really want. Though it may have the same effect.

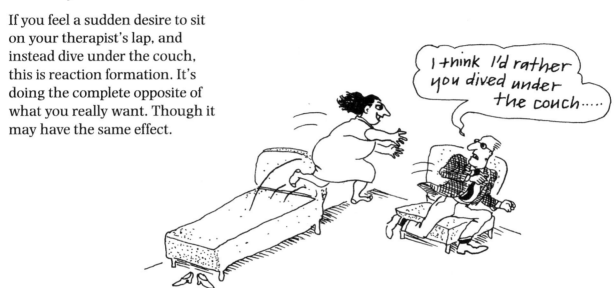

Resistance

You know you've hit resistance when your mind goes blank, or you can't describe what's come into it. This is a signal that you've reached a crucial point of anguish. You just have to hang in there until it gets resolved.

It's either a crucial point of anguish — or radishes....

Interpretation

At last the therapist lays her cards on the table and says what she thinks is really going on. This, she hopes, will lead you to insight; to find meaning where you couldn't see it; to get back feeling.

It is up to you to say whether it makes sense to you or not.

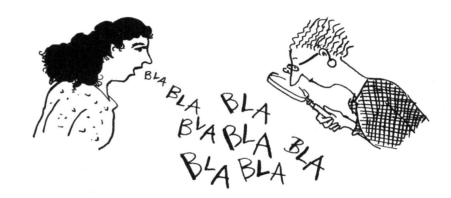

Acting in/Acting out

If you perform a somersault or sweep the photographs from your therapist's desk, you may be accused of acting in (the session). If you have an affair with a sumo wrestler whilst on holiday, this is most likely to be acting out. You will be told that there is certainly attention-seeking involved.

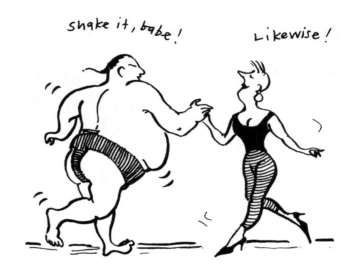

54

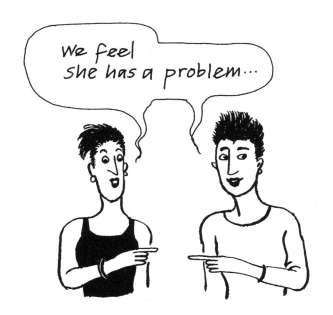

Respecting boundaries

Some couples have lived so long together that they resemble one another (the same goes for people and their pets). If you lose your boundaries – beware. Therapists are quick to point out the loss of sense of self involved.

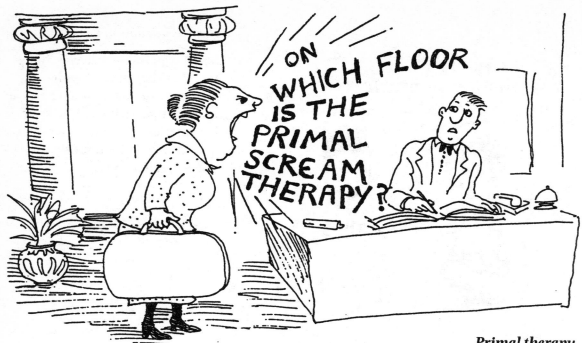

Some More Recent Therapies

Primal therapy

Primal scream therapists, of whom there are many in Southern California, have a strict routine. They may demand that you check into a hotel for three weeks.

You must agree to abstain from all drugs and tension-reducing diversions. You must then give yourself over entirely to treatment for the duration.

The aim is to get you to express your deepest feelings towards your parents. After three weeks of this intense phase you return to normal (?) life and continue treatment with a Primal Group. This therapy is not recommended to those of a suggestible disposition or with fragile lungs.

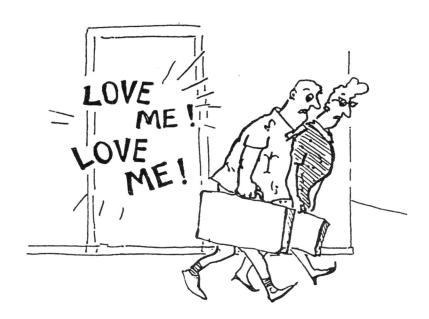

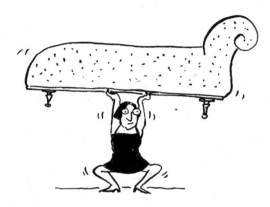

Feminist therapy

Feminist therapists recognize that in a male-dominated society women's life experiences are both different from and defined by those of men. They question or find alternatives to sexist theory, developing instead interpretations that reveal the attitudes and subtle messages which make women feel de-valued and forced to conform to male stereotypes. The aim of the therapy is to help women not only to change, but to feel empowered to lead their own lives in their own way – with or without men.

Feminist therapy has been especially helpful to women with low self-esteem, who have often been brought up to be anxious to please others. Feminist therapists are unlikely to regard lesbian or gay clients as in need of a 'cure'. But such therapy may not be to the taste of someone who regards herself as a natural wife, mother and home-maker. And it is sometimes taken to extreme lengths, especially in the USA. After all, not everyone is keen on learning to love 'the little girl within'.

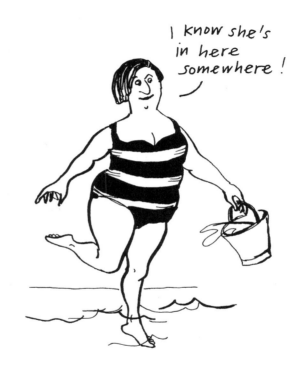

Family therapy

Freud confessed that he was 'utterly at a loss' to know how to treat patients' relatives. The answer now is often to invite the whole family into therapy. A sign that a family is not functioning properly may be that they don't communicate and there is a submerged build-up of conflict, depression, anger and resentment. This may lead to one member having an eating problem, or being cast as the scapegoat.

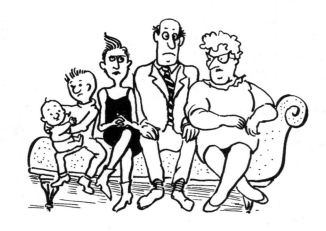

While one therapist works with the family, a second may observe the session using a one-way mirror. A feminist perspective may help by putting the family in a social context and exploring issues of gender and power. Without blaming anyone, the therapist's role is to try to help the family function in a healthier way.

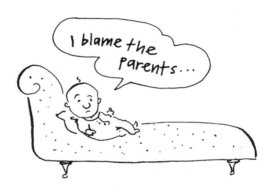

Person-centred therapy

A therapist who insists that you are the one to know which problems are crucial is likely to be a disciple of American therapist Carl Rogers. Notable for his optimistic view of human nature, he advises that a particular kind of listening called unconditional positive regard, and non-possessive warmth, be used. By respecting and valuing you, a Rogerian therapist aims to help you discover and fulfil your own potential. Rather than offering an interpretation, the therapist may reflect back to you what you say. This technique may be effective, but could be irritating.

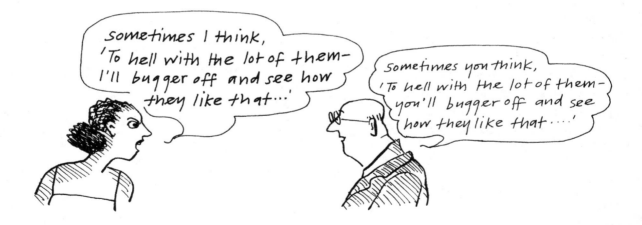

Gestalt

Developed by Fritz and Laura
Perls in the early 1950s, Gestalt
is a 'holistic' therapy. Focusing on
the need for a healthy functioning of the whole organism, it
aims to integrate body, feelings
and intellect. What is important
for the therapist is what she can
feel, see, hear and smell about
you rather than what she thinks
or interprets.

If you want to explore, experience
and discover your own shape,
pattern and wholeness, Gestalt
will enable you to integrate all
the different parts of yourself,
thus letting you become totally
what you already are, and what
you potentially can become.
Is that clear?

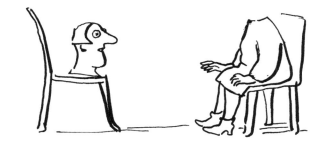

Co-counselling

A kind of double-act therapy, where two people alternately act as therapist and client. You take it in turns to relive and play out problems or traumatic events, working through negative and painful emotions which will hopefully lead to insight and emotional growth.

This is unlikely to be the best approach for someone in crisis, who may not have enough energy to put into someone else's problems.

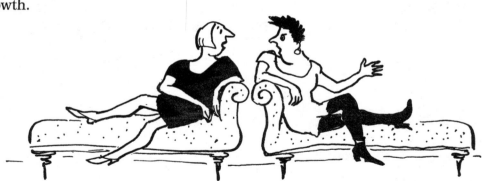

Group therapy

An alternative to individual
therapy is to meet regularly as
part of a group. Eight people
with a good therapist in a safe
place can witness and experience
such common family feelings
as hostility, envy and rivalry,
hopefully alternating with
bonding, concern and support.

Being part of a group can help to
test out irrational beliefs about
other people, and try out ways of
coping with their strange ideas
about you. It can be a useful
experience if you are shy or
withdrawn; not so good if you
feel you need a therapist to
yourself.

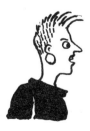

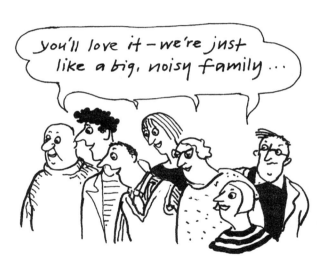

Rolfing

Photographs apparently show that rolfees grow by at least half an inch after ten bodywork sessions. This is achieved by deep massage and manipulation of the muscles to release the physical and emotional trauma that is stored there. American biochemist Dr Ida P. Rolf discovered the technique when treating her children's piano teacher's injured hand with muscle-stretching yoga exercises. She developed a theory of structural integration in which the body is seen as a series of blocks which can get unaligned.

Rolfing, the attempt to restore the body's natural equilibrium, is an acutely painful process and best avoided by those with a low pain threshold.

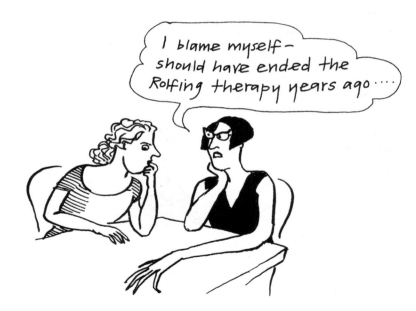

Mobile therapy

Busy executives in New York can now summon a mobile therapy van complete with chauffeur, therapist, couch, coffee table and clock. This service costs a mere $175 a session, only twice the cost of a static one.

This is not actually such a new idea. It follows in the august tradition of Freud, who used to practise mobile therapy with one of his patients on horseback.

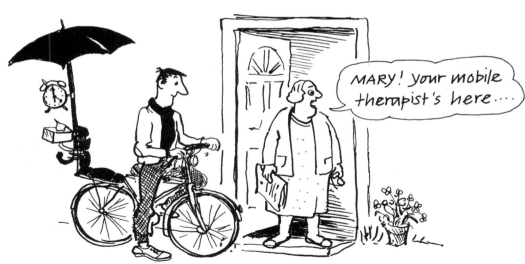

MARY! your mobile therapist's here....

OKness

Believe it or not, this really is a concept and is central to Transactional Analysis (TA). There are three not-OK positions: I'm OK – You're not OK (paranoid); I'm not OK – You're OK (depressive); I'm not OK – You're not OK (schizoid). The one to aim for is I'm OK – You're OK, a satisfactory state of existential OKness for all.

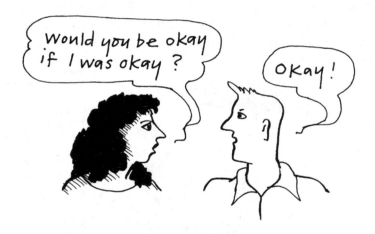

Some Behavioural and Cognitive Terms

Obsessive-compulsive disorder

Do you feel an uncontrollable need to wash your hands every 10 minutes, or to sterilize the crockery and cutlery every time you go out for a meal? If so, you are in the grip of an obsessive-compulsive disorder. This may be cured by exposure therapy, which helps you face the fears that lead to the compulsion.

Could Lady Macbeth perhaps have benefited from this technique?

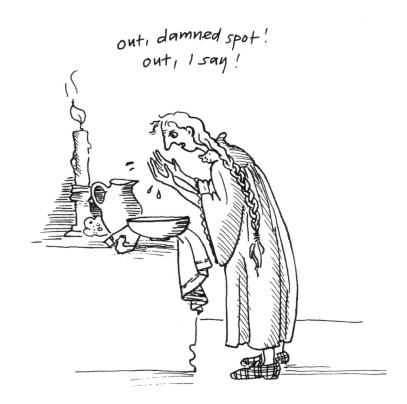

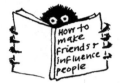

Desensitization

If you suffer from arachnophobia (fear of spiders) – or any other kind of animal phobia – it's worth giving this therapy a try.

After being shown how to relax, you will be asked to visualize a spider next to you – first a small one, then a larger one and finally something like a tarantula. When you can manage this without panic, the imaginary spider will be replaced by the genuine article. This will be brought progressively closer to you until you can hold it yourself. It may take many sessions to reach this objective.

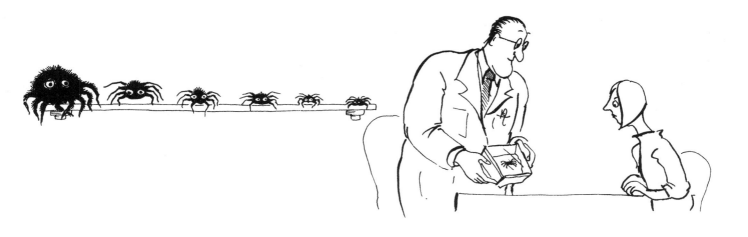

Hypnotherapy

Do you want a quick way to get in touch with your unconscious mind? Do you want to be able to switch on your own immune system? Hypnotherapy is recommended for most phobias, including fear of flying, and for sleeplessness.

After being put into a light trance state and told how to deal with the problem, you are shown how to induce this state in yourself. Contrary to popular belief, you will not have to submit yourself to the therapist's will, or turn into a zombie.

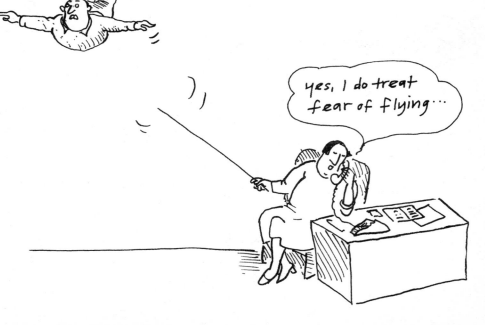

yes, I do treat fear of flying...

Neuro-linguistic programming

If you want a speedy way to give up smoking, this may be your best chance. First, the problem will be analysed from every angle. Then the therapist will try to help you change the old patterns connected with the need for a cigarette and give you alternative tasks to block out the craving.

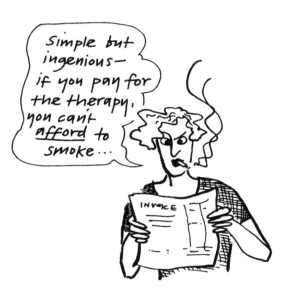

Rational-emotive therapy (RET)

RET aims to make you aware of your irrational beliefs and how they lead to unhelpful emotional states. You then learn systematically to change them. You may have to undertake specific assignments, such as a 'shame-attacking' exercise. The aim is to make you feel good about yourself even while you are carrying out a shameful act. This might mean going to Harrods and stripping to your bikini in the food hall.

Counteracting anhedonia

This is a helpful method if you are suffering from lack of pleasure. The therapist will enable you to go into a situation that you will enjoy, such as a gig, concert, rave, or Harrods food hall. Don't wear your bikini.

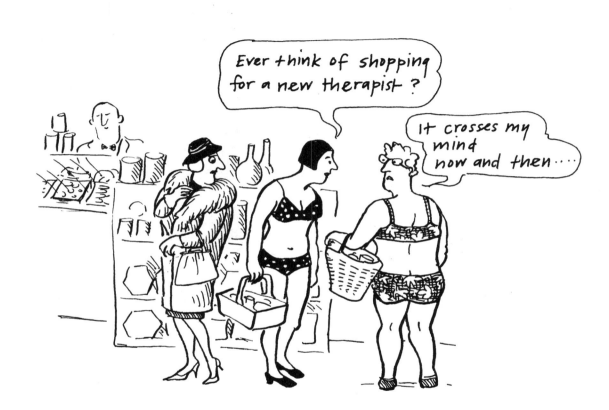

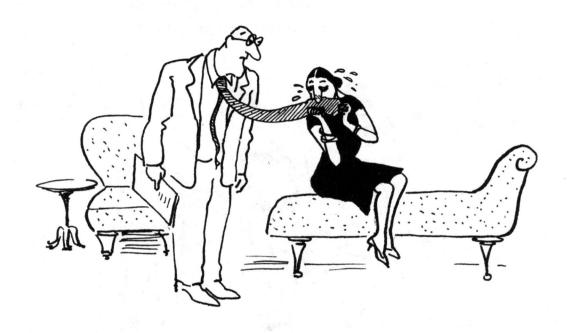

Difficult Stages to Get Through

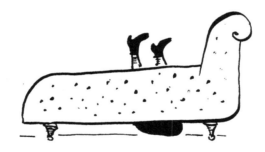

Getting through therapy is – let's be honest – a traumatic experience. In such an emotional skirmish you can be sure that anything that can go wrong, will go wrong.

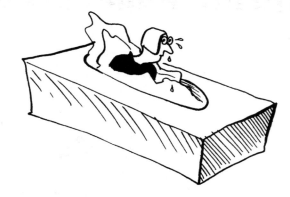

You keep forgetting to go

This resistance will be analysed. Selective memory is always suspect. It may mean that you should find another therapist or, more positively, that you need to buy a reliable alarm clock.

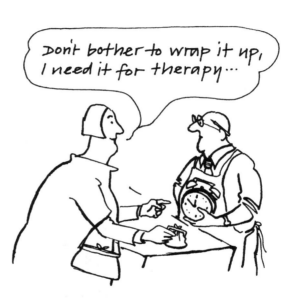

You can't go

Finding yourself in the pub at the crucial time for more than three sessions in a row may also be a reason to find another therapist. Alternatively, you could try inviting your therapist to join you there for a drink.

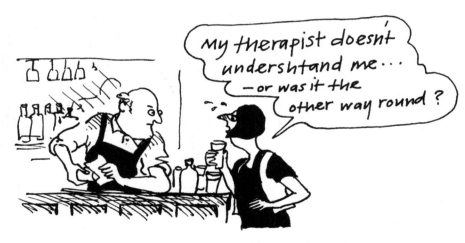

My therapist doesn't undershtand me... – or was it the other way round?

You mistake the session time

If you knock on the door and are greeted by your therapist's children, best not try to renegotiate the appointment there and then. Just beat a hasty retreat.

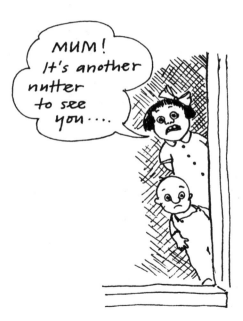

You have problems keeping appointments

Did your mother keep you waiting for half an hour every day when she picked you up from school? This may lead to problems with managing time, and even to chronic procrastination.

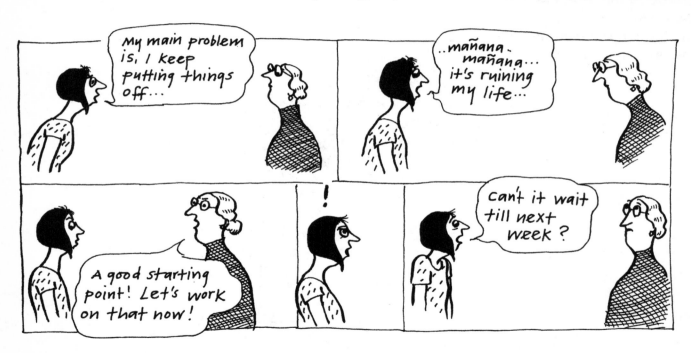

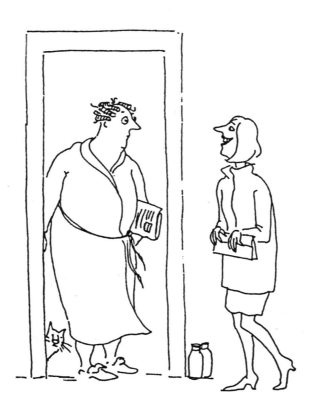

You are early and your therapist greets you in her dressing gown

Offering to make her a cup of tea will not mend the situation. Best to apologize profusely and take a turn around the block.

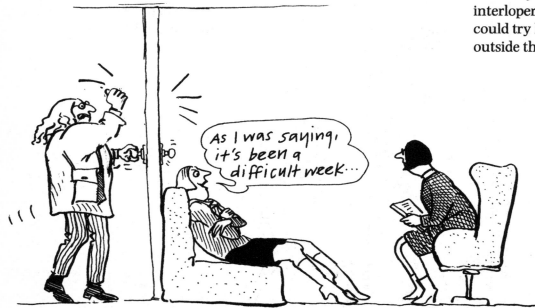

The next client keeps arriving early

Pushing an armchair against the door may help to deter would-be interlopers. As a last resort you could try leaving a large clock outside the therapy room.

You experience insatiable curiosity about your therapist

If your sessions take place in some anonymous rented room, this is unlikely to be satisfied. If you are in the therapist's home, a judicious trip to the bathroom can produce rich pickings. But beware, a flowery net cover on the spare toilet roll can produce a unique moment of truth. Lapses of memory are forgivable, but lapses of taste?

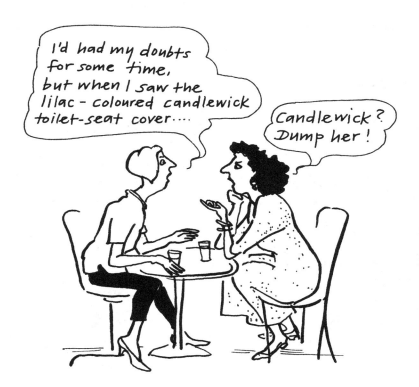

***Your therapist calls you by your
ex-partner's name***

If this happens at the end of a
session without possibility of
explanation, it can cause an
acute identity crisis.

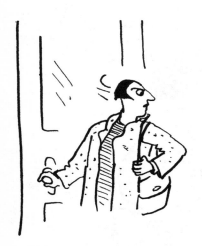

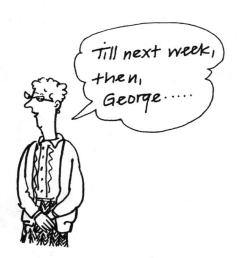

The couch has changed places with the chair

A therapist who moves her furniture around is certainly making a big statement which will get all her clients on their toes. Don't take it personally.

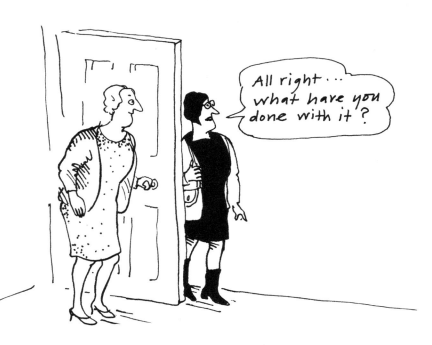

All right... what have you done with it?

Your therapist has a hot flush

The best rule of thumb is: if she would ignore your bandage, you should ignore her flush. Otherwise, offer to open the window.

You have a hot flush

Best not to start stripping off without some warning, or an alarm bell may be rung.

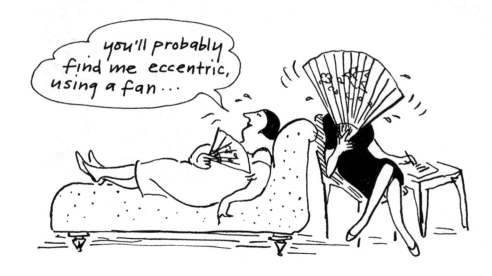

Your parents or partner want to join your session

Therapy envy is little understood by the general public. If your dear ones are too pressing, or start phoning your therapist, suggest they find their own.

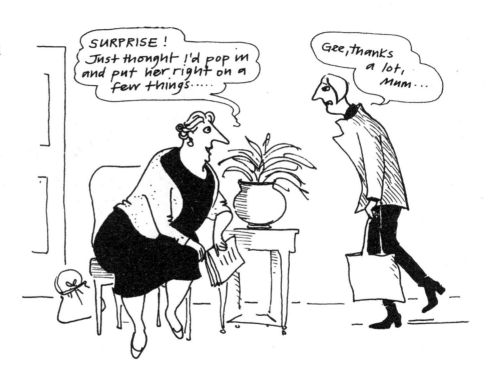

You fall in love with your therapist

This is quite common and is an opportunity to examine your projections. Don't succumb to the temptation to steal your therapist's flannel from the bathroom. This can produce complications on the home front.

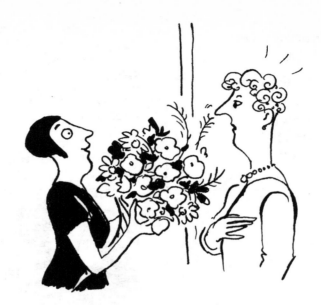

Your therapist falls in love with you

In this case you should take the initiative and suggest another look at the countertransference situation. If invited to sit on the knee, or worse, contact their professional association and seek guidance.

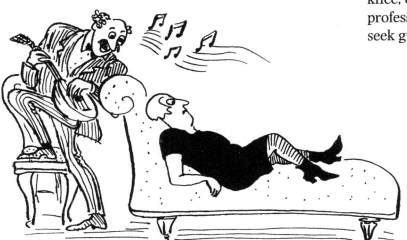

You hate your therapist and want to leave

More projections again? They will almost certainly produce an interpretation. Work through these properly before you make up your mind. Also, beware, this is the time when you are most likely to kick your therapist's dachshund or back into her car.

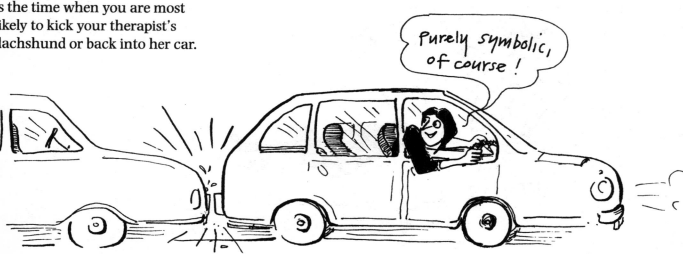

Your therapist falls asleep

This is disgracefully common, and one reason why therapists may prefer to have clients out of vision on a couch. If there is a long silence, check if you still have their attention. A persistent cough is useful here. The sound of snores will call for stronger action.

You discover you have a Royal Rival

You arrive at your session to find the building surrounded by photographers. It appears that you share your therapist with an erstwhile member of the Royal Family and the press has just found out.

Try to resist the temptation to recover your therapy fees by charging £10,000 for an exclusive interview with a tabloid.

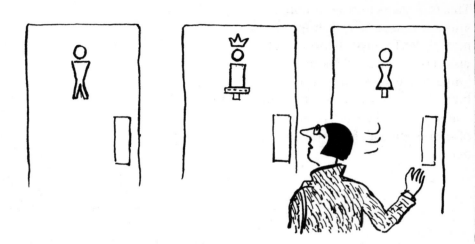

A holiday is announced

There is a general feeling that therapists should never take holidays, since, after all, they spend the whole time sitting down. If a break of any sort is looming, your therapist is likely to make a big fuss about preparing for it. It will almost certainly be suggested that any bad mood on your part is related to the forthcoming separation. Better not disabuse them of this.

Don't expect a postcard.

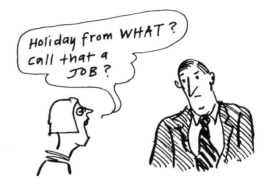

You decide to start a new relationship

All major decision-making is frowned on while therapy is in progress. At best it will be considered acting out. At worst your projections may be getting mixed up with your introjections.

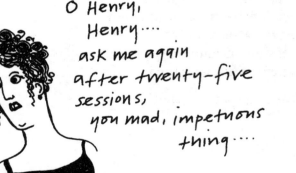

You find yourself behind your therapist in the cinema

A meeting between therapist and client in a public place can be shocking for both. Therapists have been known to hide behind pillars, supermarket trolleys and spouses in order to avoid clients. If you see a woman crouched down in her seat before the lights go up in a north London cinema, it is most likely to be some paranoid therapist undergoing a projection of her own.

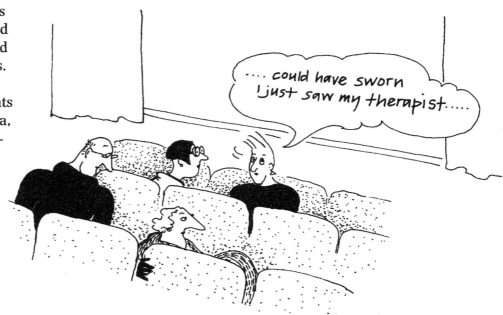

.... could have sworn I just saw my therapist .....

Telling your therapist you got drunk with her mother at a party

Coming upon a relative of your therapist in any situation is tricky. The temptation to demand to know all should be weighed against the reparation you will have to make in the next session.

You arrive drugged or drunk

This will certainly be considered to be acting out. Don't.

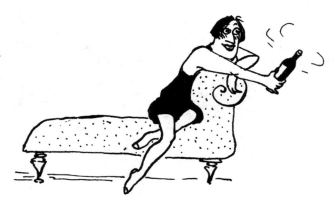

Your therapist is not there

This is devastating to even the toughest ego. No excuse should be accepted and two free sessions should be sought to work through the trauma.

Your mobile phone rings in the middle of the session

Such one-upwomanship will require major interpretation and will distract from other matters at hand. Best to switch it off beforehand.

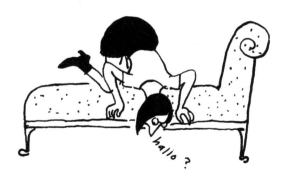

A pizza is delivered

Could this be sabotage by your
jealous partner? How your
therapist deals with the situation
will tell you a lot about the
prospects for a successful out-
come to your therapy.

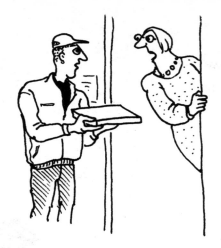

Reaching the Terminus

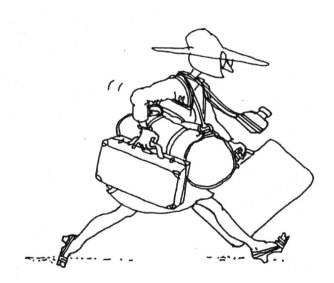

At some point, it may be after months, it may be after years, you or your therapist, or preferably both, will recognize that you have achieved as much as you probably can in your therapeutic relationship.

Alternatively, you may discover your therapist is leaving town, retiring, or emigrating to Australia.

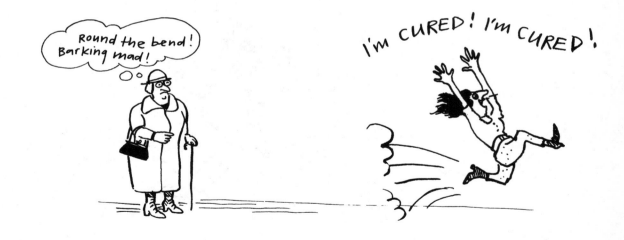

Freud believed therapy was successful when the patient had been enabled 'to work and to love', or when 'hysterical misery' was transformed into 'ordinary unhappiness'.

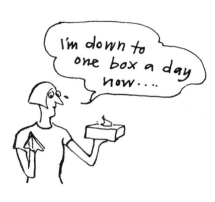

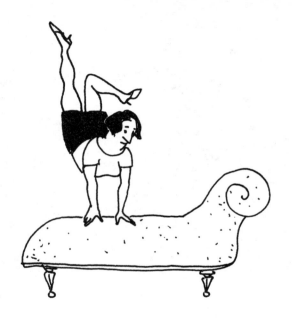

Jung thought the analyst's business was 'to help the patient towards that state where he can discover for himself the way to live and the necessary impetus to put this into practice. Theories and methods are only aims towards this end.'

According to Carl Rogers, the
client who improves 'increasingly
trusts and values the process'
which is herself. She drops the
false self, and is able to move
'away from façades'.

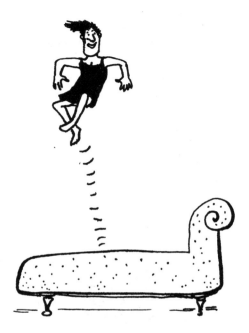

The termination process is almost always painful. It's rather like leaving home for the first time. Part of you is desperate to leave, but what will you do with your dirty washing?

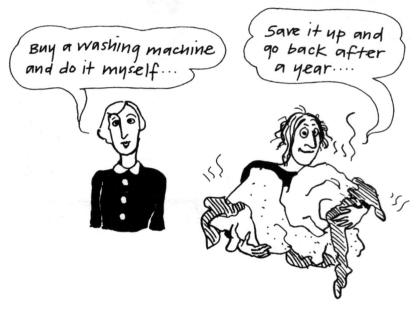

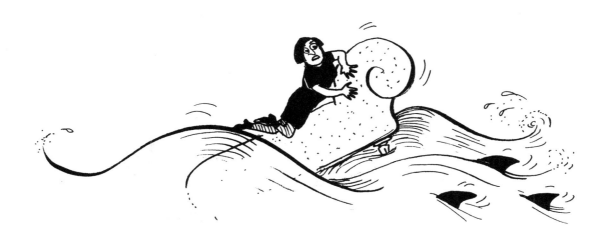

It may produce primitive fears of separation and abandonment. You may feel a strong desire to kill off the therapist before she has time to do the same to you.

Strange imagery, such as setting off on a camel down a lonely road, and the reliving of the birth process, also frequently occurs.

If you want your therapy to go on for ever, you've probably become too dependent on your therapist. Perhaps you've had too much advice instead of encouragement to seek your own answers to problems.

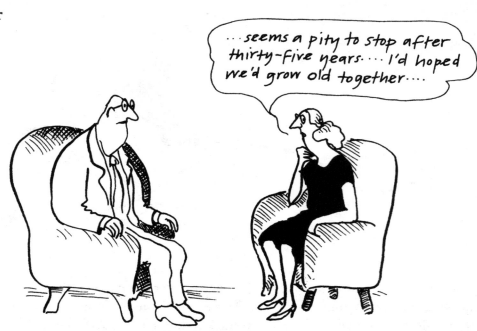

...seems a pity to stop after thirty-five years.... I'd hoped we'd grow old together....

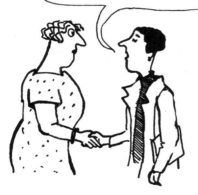

Don't keep on going because you're afraid of upsetting your therapist, fantasizing that she can't manage without you. There are plenty more where you came from.

You may find you're going to have to leave whether you like it or not because the money runs out, or your NHS sessions are up. In that case try checking out how strong you are by asking for free sessions until you're really ready to go.

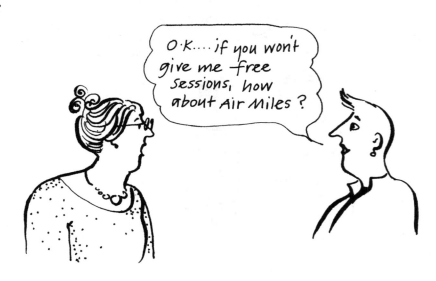

However it comes about, it is generally agreed that termination must not be hurried. It must be prepared for to allow you to give vent to all those feelings you have learnt to express so freely: anger, separation anxiety, guilt, grief and – hopefully – relief.

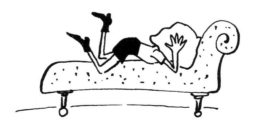

Your therapist is only human. She may appreciate a parting gift such as a poem, a bunch of flowers, a letter of thanks – or a portfolio of paintings made during the period of therapy.

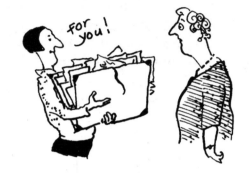

One client asked for a signed
photograph of her therapist
which she could see every day
as a substitute.

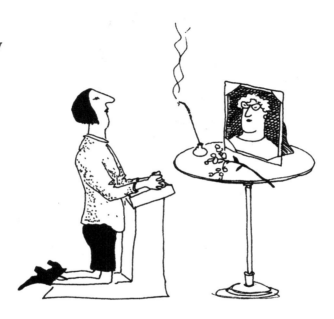

It is courteous to tell your
therapist when you have finally
had enough.

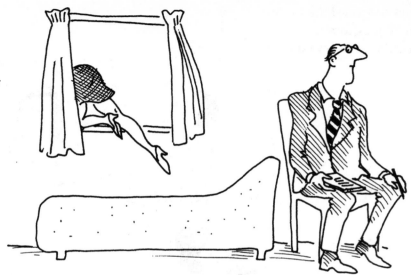

Some Alternatives to Therapy

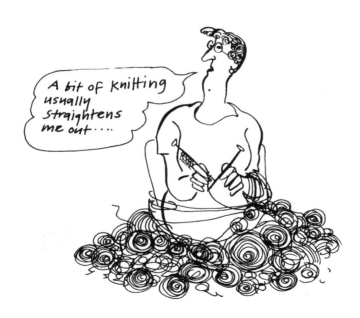

Yes, there are alternatives…

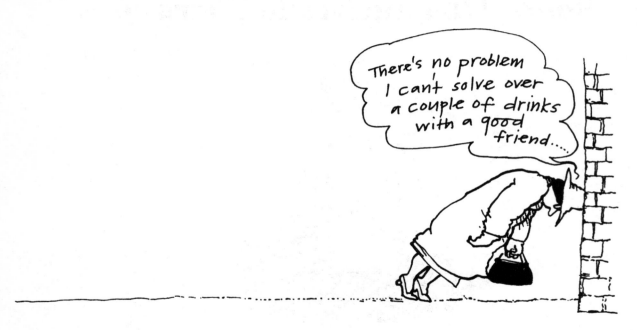

Retail therapy

Also known as repetition compulsion (or would have been if Freud had understood shopping). It is however possible to spend even more on this therapy than on the person-to-person kind and, rather than insights, to be left with a blinding overdraft.

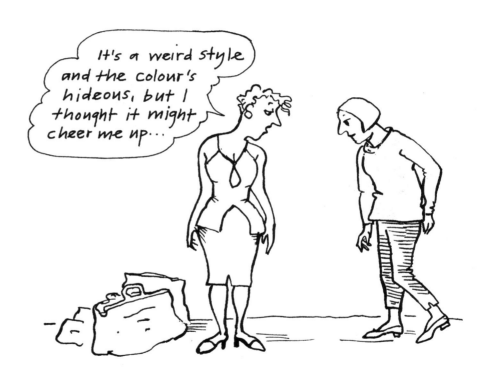

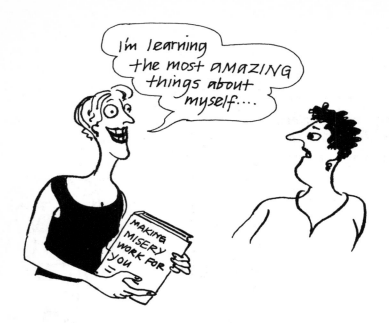

Self-help

There are any number of books, mostly written in the USA, which promote the idea that you can be your own therapist. All you need to do is think positively rather than negatively, love yourself enough, and affirm your right to be successful. What happens if you don't achieve the impossible is rarely discussed.

Cultivating your garden

The feel of soil beneath the fingernails (displacement), the sight of green shoots (projection), the pleasure of a colour-coordinated hanging basket (sublimation), these can all be satisfactory substitutes for the weekly session.

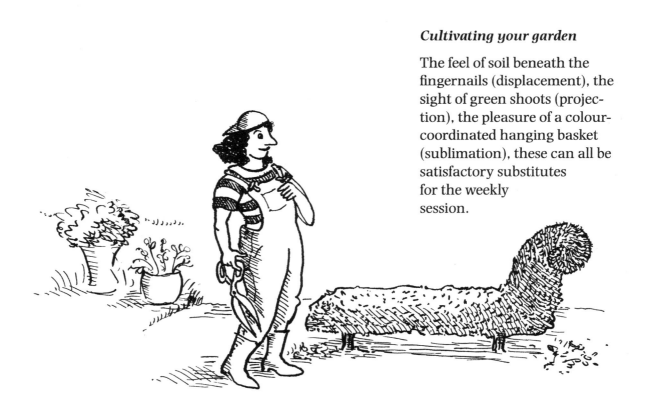

Getting a pet

Pet-keeping is now widely recognized as therapeutic for all age groups. Unlike therapists, animals have to be fed, groomed and possibly exercised. But remember that, like therapists, they need a lot of time, energy and attention; they need to be kept amused, taken care of when you go on holiday, and are mostly very expensive.

The answer may be to keep a therapist as a pet.

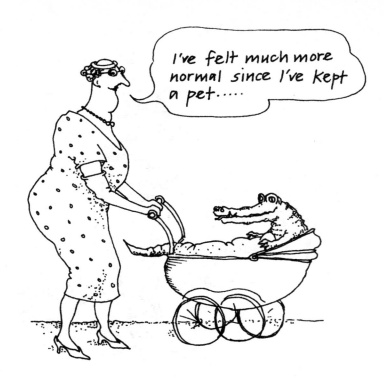

I've felt much more normal since I've kept a pet.....